AROMATHERAPY & HERBALISM

AROMATHERAPY & HERBALISM

The Complete Guide for Home Use

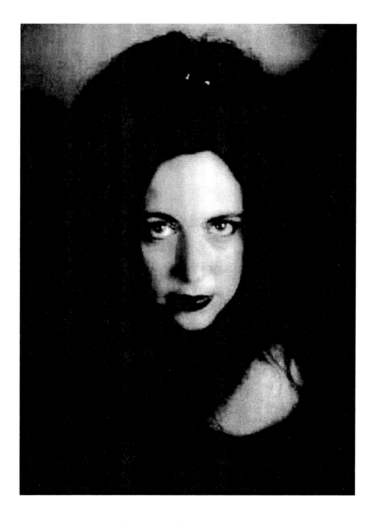

Rochelle Moore

ISBN : 1-4196-1025-2

To order additional copies, please contact us.
BookSurge, LLC
www.booksurge.com
1-866-308-6235
orders@booksurge.com

AROMATHERAPY & HERBALISM

Introduction — Smells & Spells

Once upon a time it was all so easy. If you wanted a person to fall head-over-heels in love with you, off you went to your garden, local forestry or woodland, gathered the necessary herbs or flowers and made up a recipe which ensured the final outcome would be wonderful. Likewise, if you wanted to put a curse on someone, slightly confuse or harm them, all the necessary ingredients were readily supplied by Mother Nature. In general, most people used herbs and aromas for healing purposes. They would make healing sachets for protection, for treating a psychological disorder, treat chest disorders and problem warts. However, the power of both herbs and flowers were used by some for evil purposes. The dreaded Belladonna (Atropa belladonna) is the herb that most people associate with witchcraft and magic. Other names for Belladonna are Dwale or Baneworth, this was used for flying ointments and for deadening pain. During the time of the burning anyone associated with witchcraft, Belladonna was used by the victim and swallowed so that they could pass onto the next life with as little pain as possible. Later on in the book I will show you some of the more ancient uses for herbs and include how to make flying ointment.

It was the use of herbs such as Belladonna and aromas that led to a general terror amongst the public. They were so intimidated by naturists, herbalists and aromatherapists that eventually, anyone even slightly associated with their use, were burned at the stake. However, aromatherapy and herbalism has been used by people since time began. This is an ancient and sometimes very secretive knowledge passed down through generations by wise sages, witches, shamans, doctors and right up to today's modern aromatherapists and herbalists. Many people lost their lives due to their beliefs in helping others. Their ancient knowledge was once well known by the ordinary person who could determine one herb from another, make up their own recipes and cure themselves. These ordinary people knew how to use a specific herb to ward off evil, a flower that produced sleep for those with insomnia and a combination of both to fight off many physical and psychological ailments.

Witches, naturists, alchemists, shamans, magicians, doctors and ordinary folk, all used herbs and aromas which grew abundantly in the rich meadows, alongside streams, in vast forests and in smaller woodlands locally. Many other shamans and astrologers looked to the stars for divination and for future telling. From the beginning of time right up to today, some feel it necessary to attend psychics, fortune tellers and mediums, in order to have a look into their future or receive news from their dearly departed. Today we seem to have a need to return to the older ways. With our lives constantly on the move and a world which seems to be everchanging we are once again beginning to search for the truth of our inner being. At one time most folk could fix up a remedy in a matter of minutes but, as time moved on, people became more worldly and this ancient lore was used by less and less people. Those who did keep the ancient secrets of the earth and Mother Nature alive were greatly feared and during the time of the burning, anybody slightly associated with the use of herbs or aromatherapy, were greatly feared. Those who did not die were forced into hiding or ostracised from society. Many of the older ancient secrets were lost forever with those who were burned alive. Their only crime being their belief in assisting humankind and the animal kingdom with the natural resources provided by Mother Nature.

Fewer people were interested in learning these ancient secrets due to the hideous outcome that awaited those who practised the ancient natural ways. For many years these secrets remained with a few and were highly protected and untouched. This book is my tribute to those who forfeit their lives unjustly in an attempt to nurture and retain the wisdom that, generation upon generation of wise people, had learned directly from Mother Nature herself. It is very fortunate for us today that not all was lost and that a few kept this way of life alive. It is also fortunate that there is now a great resurgence of interest by ordinary people in the protection of our planet and environment. We are now aware of just how fragile our planet really is and are actively involved in recycling, have a real interest in our health and an awareness, especially of chemical substances and food additives, which we are now turning away from and are actively seeking natural remedies for ailments—physical, emotional and psychological.

We are tired of artificial chemicals in the preparation and sale of our foods and are actively seeking natural and nourishing alternatives. People are now very aware of E numbers and foods that contain too much salt or additional additives for flavouring or appearance. The time of the ancient and natural ways are now being eagerly researched on a daily basis to improve our quality of life. In this book I shall show you how to use recipes (spells) for physical illness, emotional distress and psychological imbalance. The physical conditions covered in the book are briefly, change of life, coughs, colic, childbirth, circulation, abcesses, stings, throat problems, allergies, asthma, baldness,indigestion, migraine, nausea, neuralgia, bruises, overweight, periods, warts, rheumatism, burns and joint or muscular pains. The emotional and psychological conditions covered in the book are briefly, addictions, insomnia, hypertension, stress, anxiety, apathy, clarity, turmoil, shock, claustrophobia, trantrums,confidence, worry, courage, depression, exhaustion, fear, grief, hysteria, irrational thoughts, mental calmness or stimulation, nerves, paranoia, panic attacks and relaxation. All of the above ailments can be helped, if not cured, by simple aromatherapy and herbalism.

I am also going to show you how to easily source the herbs and essential oils that are necessary for home use via the internet, local health shops, your own garden or via post. All of the ingredients for either herbal spells or aromatherapy are easily obtainable and I have tried to keep this book as simple as possible to guide you through the use of them. This is an introduction to the use of aromas and herbal spells and I will show you how to locate, dry and prepare herbs. I will also show you how to use and combine essential oils so that you can practise this ancient craft in the comfort of your own home. A list of tools required will be outlined and towards the end of the book a few ancient secrets will be shown. I will even show you how to grow a herb wheel at home in your garden. To grow and pick your own fresh herbs is so satisfying and also the herbs are three times more potent than that purchased in the supermarket. The techniques for making sachets, poultices, scented oiles, incenses, amulets and infusions are shown clearly. None of the enclosed techniques are impractical and all can be used within your daily life. Whether you wish to simply make up an aphrodisiac, overcome panic attacks, attract love and passion, aid fertility or bring personal happiness into your lives, you can choose which way you wish to go and enjoy this ancient craft. I shall briefly touch off on other areas such as meditation, personal happiness, great health and the development of your inner being to it's fullest potential.

Your sense of smell is one of your most powerful of all senses. Ancient sages burned herbs on open fires to induce the required effect. During the plague in England in the 17th century, essential oils were used to ward off this lethal illness. The secretive ancient ways can be used in your daily life for a better understanding of yourself, a better standard of living and will bring your mind, body and spirit together in complete harmony. You are so much more than you think and I hope to show you how to create a wellbeing, beauty, flowing harmony and a completeness of expression that will change the way you perceive yourself. All thoughts, acts and deeds are a part of you that can be used to open up a new door and guide you down the pathway to complete happiness. Love & light.

Contents
WHAT IS AROMATHERAPY AND HERBALISM?

This section of the book contains the names of aromatherapy oils, the use of herbs, how to obtain and care for essential oils and herbs, the purchase of oils, how long the amulets and oils will last, a list of essential oils and how to use them. Oils and herbs can be used for mental stress, physical ailments, for spritual or mood enhancing and for what some may consider, supernatural purposes. Most essential oils are easily located at your local supermarket, health store or via the internet. The basic herbs required for use are provided by Mother Nature and are also easily obtained. In part of of this book I shall show you how to select, gather, dry and store nature's herbs. I shall also outline the list of tools that you will require and where they can be sourced. There will be a list and and easy reference guide to ailments, psychological, spiritual and physical. I will show you the extreme strength of essential oils and herbs and point out the specific cases in which they cannot be used.

SMELLS & SPELLS

This part of the book will show you how to use and how to make up spells and oils. For some ailments only one type of remedy will be shown, aromatherapy or herbalism, as you will only need the one type for success. I will clearly show you in an easily followed step-by-step guide how to make up some of the ancient recipes which have been kept a secret for so many years. I will outline the more powerful aromatherapy and herbal potions of which many are thousands of years old. I will show you how to make oils for massage, inhalers, compresses, room fragrancers, perfumes and mood enhancing aromas. On the same page, I will show you how to use herbs for the same purposes. Some oils cannot treat certain ailments so I shall show you the herbal remedy and vice-versa.

I Would Like To Dedicate This Book To Shaun And Kyle. Through Their Youthful Eyes I Have Seen So Many Aspects And Perceptions Of The Way Our Life Should Be. I Can Never Express In Words My Absolute And All Encompassing Love And Dedication That I Have For These Two Beautiful People. Thank You Both For Showing Me Just How True Love, With No Boundaries, Realy Feels.

Old remedies & Secrets

In the final part of this book I will show you recipes that are thousands of years old. Here you will find anything from wand making to flying ointment. I would like to thank and pay a tribute to those brave people who managed to keep these ancient secrets throughout the generations, many of whom died for their belief in helping mankind and the animal kingdom. I hope you enjoy this step-by-step introduction to the use of aromatherapy and herbalism. Please remember that any of the spells in this book should only be used for good purposes and never on anybody who is not aware of your intentions.

"As if a cloud has been raised from your vision, begin to discover your true identity. You will begin to see life from the perspective of the ancient natural ways. Your buried interests in oils and herbs will be awakened. Appeciate your natural environment and see the beauty of nature through happy and appreciative eyes. If you feel depressed, angry or irritable, you do not have to make many radical life changes, just use flowers, oils and inner truth to find the true inner you. You have the choice through your thoughts, emotions, intentions and choice of direction to make your life complete. Sometimes we are not even aware of the detrimental impact of stress in our life. All around moves fast and sometimes our system can become overloaded. Deep down you know the type of life you want to live. You deserve the best in life and with Mother Nature's natural assistance, you can achieve it.

You will be amazed at the accuracy of the enclosed information. It is up to you to clarify your way and make the decision on which herbs or oils are best suited to your particular needs. No matter how inexperienced you are you will achieve positive results. With practise, you will come to use your own personal interpretation and select the remedies best suited to you. Another important aspect within your lives is colours which i will show you on the next page. At the end of the book I will show you a wonderful array of superstitions both bizzare and real. I wish you great health and happiness—have fun.

The Meaning of Colours

Just as aromas and herbs can influence your mood so can colours. You can select a room colour, burn coloured candles, burn incenses or select any of the below for mood altering purposes:-

WHITE—Work, blessing, purity and giving

BLACK—Banishing illnesses, breaking curses and can be oppresive

BROWN—Creating a healing environment for animals

PURPLE—Boosting your spiritual awareness

BLUE—Healing, peace and scerenity

RED—Passion, lust and vitality

YELLOW—Stimulation of your mental powers

GREEN—Fertility and prosperity

PINK—Affection, true love and healing

PEACH—Calming and healing

CREAM -Freedom if used sparingly

LILAC—Spirituality

SILVER—Inner space

GREY—Diversity

CERISE—Spirituality and love

GOLD—Spirituality

VIOLET—Highest spiritual colour

INDIGO—Intuition, beauty and poetic

Colours Effects on your Body & Mind

RED—Lower spine and genital area. This colour is physical, strong, extrovert, passionate, physical love, energetic, generous and sensuous. If your favourite colour is red then you are a great lover of life, balanced and harmonious.

YELLOW—The solar plexus. This colour is forgiveness, courage, forward going, intellectual, inspirational and full of variety. If your favourite colour is yellow then you are lively, love nature, sunny, full of variety and courage.

BLUE—The throath. This colour is a heavenly and healing colour. It depicts tranquility, depth of character, spirituality and freedom. If your favourite colour is blue then you are extremely versitile, relaxed, a very deep thinker and you strive for knowledge.

GREEN—The heart. This colour is compassionate, spiritual, cosmic, lover of nature, healing and tranquil. If your favourite colour is green then you tend to put others before yourself at times. You are very down to earth, balanced and a natural carer.

ORANGE: Stomach and intestines. This colour is just so full of life and natural energy. It is outgoing, strong, lively, and very physical. If your favourite colour is orange then you are just bursting with natural energy and life, healthy and a great lover of tranquility.

VIOLET—Top of the head. This colour is just the most spiritual of all. It is wonderful for spirituality, inspirational, very sensitive, courage and yet sometimes withdrawn. If your favourite colour is violet then you are a very deep spiritual person, love time alone and yet can get lonely easily, courage comes when you need it and a great lover of tranquility.

INDIGO—Forehead. This colour is very spiritual and very aware of supernatural occurances. It represents many different aspects of freedom, courage, love, very intuitive and poetic. If your favourite colour is indigo then you are very aware of any supernatural energies, very wise, sensitive and creative.

General Cautions

Never use any essential oils directly onto your skin and never use them internally. During pregnancy only use half of the amount stated in the book. Keep all essential oils out of your eyes and away from children at all times. Should you accidentally get any oils into your eyes wash them out immediately with plenty of water and seek medical advice.

BABIES & INFANTS: Children from the day they are born up until six years old can only use certain recommended oils and very sparingly. Please take particular care and examine the dosage closely. The main oils that can be used on this age group are Lavender or Roman Chamomile—one drop of oil only in a bath, as a room fragrancer or as a compress.

CHILDREN & TEENS: Children from the age of seven up until the age of thirteen need to use less amounts of oils than adults. This is due to their size and it is important that you study this section closely as overuse of oils and their potency can be detrimental. The main oils that can be used for this age group is Tea Tree, Lavender or Roman Chamomile—one to three drops in a bath, for massage, in a compress or as room fragrancers.

TEENS & ADULTS: Children from the age of thirteen can use the same dosage as that for adults. All methods can be used such as inhalers, compresses, room fragrancers, massage and bathing.

PREGNANCY: During pregnancy only use the oils in half the stated doses. Special oils should be avoided completely such as: Basil, Clove, Cinnamon, Hyssop, Juniper, Marjoram, Myrrh, Sage and Thyme.

ALLERGIES & SKIN SENSITIVITY: Any person who suffers

from allergies to soaps, perfumes or flowers which cause irritation, must not use any form of stimulating oils. If you find that you are sensitive to a particular oil just smooth your base Almond Oil onto the area and it should cease within an hour or so. Do not use any oil on your skin that is an irritant.

HORMONAL CHANGES: Most women during hormonal changes can be extra sensitive to particular oils. This is common around the change or just prior or after menstruation. Just dilute the oils around this time of the month and during the change. Certain oils should be completely avoided due to the strength such as Hyssop and Sage. You should go to a qualified aromatherapist if these oils are required for any particular reason.

HOMOEPATHIC TREATMENTS: If you are currently receiving homoepathic treatments please consult your homeopath particularly about the following essential oils as they may not be suitable at this time; Black Pepper, Camphor and Eucalyptus.

TOOLS FOR AROMATHERAPY

I nhalation is a very effective way of introducing aromas into the body. This method is especially effective if you have bronchial problems, for soothing the respitory tract, nasal congestion or for breaking up catarrh. Inhalation is a simple method and all that you require is a basin, warm water and the wise old method of placing a towel over your head. Make sure that the water is not too hot as this can burn up the oils before you get any benefit from them. Place a couple of drops of essential oils into the water, stir and then inhale the vapours.

Massage is a highly effective method of using aromatherapy oils. The requirements for massage include a base oil which is always used and then you add in your drops of essential oil and mix. The best base oil I have found is Almond Oil. This is a very therapeutic form of using oils and ifyou take a short course in the basics of massage it is highly informative and will help you along this road swiftly.

Diffusion is another highly effective method for introducing aromatherapy into your home. This is such a popular method that most commercial companies are mass producing items that emit fragrances in various ways. However, there is nothing as satisfying and personal as the making up of your own particular fragrances. You can select them for smell only or blend together oils that will be beneficial for your particular ailments. An oil burner, candles, a few drops of water and oils is all that you require for diffusion.

Compresses can be used for stings, bites, sunburn, burns or any general outer ailment. Compresses are made up of clean material, essential oils (about two drops) placed in a basin of water and then applied to the area required.

Humidifiers can be bought for regular home use. However, it is just as effective and less costly to place a saucer of water with a few drops of essential oil on top of a radiator which will act as a home-made humidifier or vapouriser. If you have insomnia, you can place a little water into a saucer, put a few drops (about three) of lavender oil, mix well and put directly onto a radiator in your bedroom.

Handkerchiefs or tissues are very easily obtained and a cost effective alternative to more expensive materials. This fast method whereby you place a few drops (about two or three) of essential oils directly onto the surface is generally used during travelling. This can also be used efficiently if you do not have the toools such as incense burners or humidifiers, readily available.

Sleeves are another alternative. If you suffer from panic attacks you can place a few drops (about two) directly onto your sleeve (Lavender or Frankincense) and if you start to hyperventilate just smell directly.

Another item which you can carry at all times is Rescue Remedy as it is a wonderful mixture that can be used regularly during the day to alleviate stress, panic, fear, tension and many other forms of ailments.

TOOLS FOR HERBALISM

A Mortar and Pestle are used for grinding up of herbs, bark or flowers. They are essential for mixing of incenses and powders. You can purchase these in the cookery section at most supermarkets, herb stores, health stores or major department store. These items are available in various sizes and materials. Wooden Mortars and Pestals are not recommended as they can easily splinter. The most popular types are made from stone, metal or marble.

A heat resistant glass container which is two-quarts in size (a glass of beer) and not made of metal. This implement is used as a condenser and to brew infusions. Make sure that the implement used has a lid which will contain any valuable steam that the herbs emit from escaping.

Fire is the next essential tool. A gas stove, a cooker, a camping stove or an open fire is necessary for heating purposes. An open fireplace and an old cauldron is the original method of heating brews.

Candles and candle holders are essential in as many colours as possible. As outlined previously, colours can play a vital role as well as aromas. Make sure you have a good stock of multi-coloured candles on hand at all times.

A censer or an incense burner is also used to purify the area in which you make your recipe. This is an ancient way of purifying the surrounding area with the best aromas for cleansing being Frankincense or Rosemary.

Spring water is the purest when making up herbal brews. If you are lucky enough to have a natural spring nearby you can stock up on this pure water. If you do not have access to a natural spring, bottled spring water will suffice.

Pure virgin oil is required when making up most recipes or spells. Make sure that you always have an ample supply at hand when you wish to make up your brews.

For sachets or amulets always have a wide and varied selection of threads, yarns, muslin and cheesecloth. Make sure you have as many colours as possible as it is important how your sachet or amulet look.

An eye dropper is a very useful implement when blending oils or whilst making up recipes. It saves you a great amount of time and is a very accurate way to measure out exact amounts for potions.

Finally, you will need a very large stock of herbs. You can start off by buying them at your local health shop or supermarket and eventually work up to growing your own. Later on in the book I will show you just how easy it is to make your own herbal wheel. This is both a cost-effective and highly enjoyable way of supplying your own herbs.

Now that you know what is required it is time to enjoy yourself and follow the enclosed instructions closely. You can now take back control of your health and get back to Mother Nature.

STORAGE OF ESSENTIAL OILS

Essential oils can be purchased from various suppliers, health stores, department stores or online. When purchasing oils make sure that the bottle reads "pure essential oils". All oils should be stored in dark bottles in which they were supplied or if you mix up your own batch make sure to use dark glass bottles as oils are very powerful and would damage plastic containers. Keep the oils in a cool place away from the reach of children and direct sunlight. If you store your oils correctly, blended oils can last for up to two years in a cool place or a refrigerator. Certan oils such as Orange can only be stored for a period of six months.

Base oils must be of very high quality and the best of these are extra virgin cold pressed oils. One of the most popular base oils is Sweet Almond and it is widely used for many purposes.

Essential Oils you will Need

This is a list of all oils and their purposes. You can select which ones to buy that suit your own personal physical or psychological needs.

ALMOND — *Determination, energy and zest*
BASIL — *Nerves, exhaustion, headache, sinus, fertility, arguments*
BERGAMONT — *Anxiety, depression, fear, boils and stress*
BENZOIN — *Dry skin, blisters or extreme sadness*
BLACK PEPPER — *Flu, aches, constipation and fever*
CAJUPUT — *Clarity, obsession, memory and disorientation*
CARDAMON — *Indigestion, confusion of the mind or selfishness*
CEDARWOOD — *Asthma, bronchitis, stress and dandruff*
CHAMOMILE (ROMAN) — *Boils, colic, eczema and tantrums*
CINNAMON — *Flu symptoms and shivering*
CLARY SAGE — *Addiction, insomnia, stress and hyperactivity*
CLOVE — *Toothache*
CORIANDER — *Loss of appitite, love and love potions*
CYPRESS — *Bronchitis, cellulitis, dandruff, periods and jealousy*
EUCALYPTUS — *Cattrrh, runny nose, congestion and cystitis*
FENNELL — *Bloated tummy, wind, flatulence and overweight*
FRANKINCENSE — *Abscess, acne, courage and panic attacks*
GERANIUM — *Lice, hormone imbalance, PMT and mood swings*
GINGER — *Arthritis, flu and self-acceptance*
GRAPEFRUIT — *Clarity, envy and worry about the past*
HYSSOP — *Grief and hypertension*
JASMINE — *Apathy, aphrodisiac, shyness, sexual prowess and childbirth*
JUNIPER — *Cystitis, hangover, rheumatism, hay fever and cramps*
LAVENDER — *Abscess, hysteria, antibiotic, arthritis, fear of people, failure, stage fright, baldness, bedwetting, insomnia, coughs, mood swings, throat, tendons, impatience, bruises, cuts, irritability, cystitis, hyperactivity, nerves, exhaustion, flushes, overwork, swollen joints, paranoia, migraine, nausea,*

overactive mind, panic attacks, nosebleeds, pregnancy, PMT, burns, weeping skin, stings, sunbury and worry.

LEMON—Sluggishness, cellulitis, warts and verrrucas

LEMONGRASS—Boredom, insect repellent and nervous exhaustion

MARJORAM—Muscle relaxant, mental strain and hyperactivity

MELLISA—Shock, worry about the future and heavy periods

MYRRH—Dry cough

NEROLI—Stress, shock, broken veins and bereavement

ORANGE—Stubborness, marriage problems and lack of vigour

PATCHOULI—Apprehension, sores and overweight

PEPPERMINT—Mental stimulant, stomach, neuralgia and nausea

PINE—Unblocking sinus or for cold symptoms

ROSE—Love potions, passion, desire and femininity

ROSE OTTO—Addiction, hangover, PMT, regret and terror

ROSEMARY—Baldness, leathagy, memory, hangover, migraine, chilblains, circulation, muscle aches, mental stimulation, calmness, protection and tiredness

ROSEWOOD—Apprehension, stability and daydreaming

SAGE—Stimulant for the metabolism

SANDALWOOD—Recurrent dreams, failure, humility, catarrh, voice loss, sinustis, tinnitus, irritability, worry about the future and sensitivity

TEATREE—Antibiotic, mouth ulcers, thrush, veruccae and acne

THYME—Throat infections

VALERIAN—Nerves, injection passion into a stale marriage and stress

YLANGYLANG—Anger, aphrodisiac, guilt, jealousy, impatience, irritability, panic attacks, self esteem, self confidence, shyness, sensitivity, stubbornness and suspicion

Identifying, storage and drying herbs
MAKING UP TINCTURES AND INFUSIONS

Years ago people had to hunt out herbs from all sources, gather them and then dry them. Today it is a lot simpler as you can purchase most herbs from your supermarket, health store or online. Herbs which you grow or pick from the wild have three times the potency of store bought ones. If you are lucky enough to be able to go into the wild and pick your own herbs please ensure that they are not polluted by modern motorways or near stale stagnant water. Another thing to bear in mind is that the herbs have not been sprayed by chemicals or insecticides.

GATHERING HERBS

Rule number one "if you are not absolutely sure what herb you are looking at, dont pick it". The potency of herbs can easily be underestimated and results can be fatal. If you wish to use the ancient methods of herb gathering, obtain herbs as follows:-

Root crops should be picked during a waning Moon, from full to new

Flowers, leaves and all seeds should be picked during the waxing Moon, from new to full

Never pick up any flowers, leaves, seeds or root crops that have been left lying on the ground or have dark spots or patches on them. All should be fresh when picked.

DRYING HERBS AND FLOWERS

Firstly, as already stated, never use any brown, insect eaten herbs or flowers that are lying on the ground. All herbs and flowers must be fresh. If you could purchase a small book which clearly identifies herbs you will learn which herb is which. Wash all herbs and flowers in pure spring water. Make sure that all the soil or earth is completely gone. Pat them dry with a paper kitchen towel or a clean dry cloth. To dry leaves you spread them on a baking sheet. Turn the leaves daily to ensure that mould does not set in and never allow near direct sunlight. When the leaves are dry they will crumble at your touch. Pick out any stems or stalks.

To dry flowers use exactly the same method as above.

The dry seeds and seed heads you tie the stems together and place them in a paper bag. Hang the bag with the flower heads facing down so that all seeds that drop from the flowerhead will be safely retained. You can keep the paper bags in direct sunlight or near to heat as this quickens up the process. When dry, shake the bag so that all the seeds will separate from the seed heads. This is generally a very fast process.

The drying of roots is by far the longest process. The best way to dry out roots is to hang them directly beside a fire or put them into your airing cupboard. If you don't have the patience to wait for anywhere from three months up to a year, dry the roots in an oven for a few minutes. If you are using this method watch them carefully as you do not want any roots to turn brown or burn.

TINCTURES: This is the extraction of the goodness of the herb or flower by the use of alcohol. Tinctures last up to two years if stored in dark airtight glass bottles. You will need to use 4 ounces of dried herb and 2 glasses of vodka. Place in a glass jar with a tight lid and leave for two weeks. When ready, strain through a clean muslin cloth and store the tincture in dark bottles, date and label well. You can use up to 15 drops of a tincture three times a day.

INFUSIONS: Add one to two teaspoons of dried herbs (or two to four fresh herbs) to a cup of boiling water. Leave for about 10 minutes and strain through a strainer. You can drink a cup of infusion up to three times a day. It can be either hot or cold.

Sorting Herbs and Flowers

Just like essential oils, herbs prefer to be stored in dark glass bottles. A real herbalist would have a vast selection at any one time as the process for storage is an ongoing one. Each bottle must be air-tight, corked or have a secure lid on it. Before using or re-using a bottle please ensure that it is completely washed and dried. Another handy item to have at hand is a roll of labels. Write the name of the potion clearly, the date that it was bottled and any other relevant information. Herbs or flowers should be restocked every six months. By keeping your potions correctly labelled, up-to-date and in clean air-tight containers you will retain the power of the mixture for longer and avoid any unnecessary accidents.

Herbs and Flowers you will Need

As with Essential Oils you select the recipes that are most suitable for your specific requirements. Select the herbs from the list below:-

ACADIA — Meditation, spiritual and psychic powers
ACORNS — Fertility
ANGELICA — Protection and purification
ANIST — Clairvoyance and divination
APPLE — Love
ASTER — Love
AVENS — Purification
BALM OF GILEAD — Protecction, love or when love has died
BASIL — Protection and purification
BASIL MYRTLE — Love potions
BATCHELOR'S BUTTONS - Love
BAY — Purification and love
BAYBERRY — Prosperity at home and money in your pocket
BAY LAUREL — Protection
BERGAMONT — Love and mood altering
BIRCH LEAVES — Healing
CHAMOMILE (ROMAN) — Healing
CARAWAY — Love and love potions
CARNATIONS — Healing and spice up your love life
CATNIP — Love
CHICORY — When love has died
CINNAMON - Healing and love
CLOVES — Clairvoyance
COLTSFOOT — Love
CORIANDER — Love and passion
COSTMARY — Clairvoyance
CUMIN — Love

CYCLAMEN—Protection and reviving stagnant love
DILL—Protection
DRAGONS BLOOD—Love, desire and passion
ELECAMPANE—Love
ENCHINACEA—Healing
EUCALYPTUS—Healing
FENNELL—Protection
FERN—Protection
FLAX—Protection
FRANKINCENSE—Divination
GARDINEA—Peace and harmony
GARLIC—Protection, healing and anti-sickness
HAZELNUTS—Fertility
HENBANE—Love, desire and fertility
HONEYSUCKLE—Forget an ex lover
HOREHOUND—Protection
JASMINE—Love and passion
JUNIPER—Protection and purification
LADY'S SLIPPER—Protection
LEMON BALM—Love, desire, passion and clairvoyance
LAUREL—Divination
LAVENDER—Healing and love
LOTUS—Healing
LOVAGE—Love and passion
MANDRAKE—Love and sexual prowess
MARJORAM—Love
MEADOWSWEET—Love
MINT—Love and clairvoyance
MISTLETOE—Protection
MUGWORTH—Protection, purification and clairvoyance
MULLEIN—Protection
MUSK—Love, passion and desire
MYRRH—Healing
MYRTLE—Love
NARCISSUS—Healing
ONIONS—Anti-sickness and nausea
ORRIS ROOT—Love, lust and passion
PATCHOULI—Love
PEONY ROOTS—Protection
PINK GERANIUM—Love, lust and passion
PERIWINKLE—Protection and love

IMPERNEL—*Protection*
POPPY—*Fertility*
PURSLANE—*Rid yourself of hurt after a failed relationship*
ROSE—*Love*
ROSE GERANIUM—*Protection*
ROSEMARY—*Protection, purification, healing and stress*
ROSE PETALS—*Clairvoyance and love*
ROWAN—*Protection*
RUE—*Protection*
SAGE—*Healing*
SAFFRON—*Healing*
SANDALWOOD—*Healing*
SATYR OIL—*Very potent for men to attract women*
SOUTHERNWOOD—*Love, lust and passion*
ST. JOHN'S WORTH—*Protection and purification*
STRAWBERRY LEAVES—*Love*
SNAPDRAGON—*Protection*
SPEARMING—*Healing*
TANSY—*Love*
TARRAGON—*Protection*
TONKA BEANS—*Love, passion and desire*
TREFOIL—*Protection*
VALERIAN—*Love and relaxation*
VIOLET—*Healing, love, passion and lust*
VERVIAN—*Protection and love*
YARROW—*Purification and love*

Massage using Oils

The use of massage is a very soothing and relaxing way of introducing oils into your body. This is particularly suitable for people suffering from stress, overwork, panic attacks or anxiety. You can go to a qualified therapist, explain your personal situation to them, and they will use the oils that you have selected from the above list and are most beneficial for you.

If you are using the oils at home it they must be mixed with a base oil which I will show you later in the book. For the elderly, massage of the hands and feet can be very soothing and relaxing. Generally, massage should not be used on anyone who has cancer before consulting their doctor.

Bathing

Using oils in a bath is the second most effective way of introducing them into your body. The best way to use essential oils while bathing are as follows:

Run your bath with warm water. Hot water can evaporate the oils and decrease the benefit to your body. Add up to five drops of essential oils directly to your bath. You can mix the type of oils you wish to use. Stir you bath so that the oils are evenly dispersed. Totally relax for about fifteen minutes in the bath and top up with warm water if necessary. As ever, avoid getting essential oils in your eyes. If this does occur, rinse out immediately with water.

You can bathe using oils in your bath daily. The effects of the oils may work immediately or take up to 24 hours—this totally depends on the type of oils that you have slected. The usual rule of thumb is that the oils begin to work immediately.

Inhaling

Inhaling oils is a great way for relieving catarrh, congestion, for colds and general respiratory conditions. This method is very gentle and easy way of introducing oils into your body. For easing your breathing or any of the above simply place about 8 drops of Eucalyptus, or any other suitable oil, into a basin with two pints of warm water. As with the procedure for bathing, stir the water until the oils have completely mingled, cover your head with a towel and inhale the vapours. This can be repeated safely a few times a day.

Compresses

The use of compresses is so easy. If you have a first aid kit then follow the instructions. However, if you do not have a first aid kit to hand, simply select a suitable dry clean cloth, add two drops of the required oil into water, place the cloth on the surface of the water, remove after a few minutes and place the compress directly on the area that it is required.

Fragrances for Rooms

You can burn oils mixed with water in oil burners. Just fill the top of the oil burner with a little water and add 5 drops of essential oil. This can be one fragrance or you can make a blend of a couple of oils to burn. Light a candle beneath the oil burner and let the heat evaporate the water and send the fragrance around your room. Oil burners can change the atmosphere in a room within minutes creating a relaxing ambience (lavender) or another type of oil to induce whatever mood you require. Alternatively, you can purchase incense sticks to burn but I feel that it is far more beneficial and satisfying when you choose your own aromas.

Quick Solutions

If you do not have an oil burner or incense sticks readily available your can use the handiest solution for you. You could always place a few drops of oil into a small container, such as a saucer, directly onto a radiator. If someone is suffering from insomnia, select Lavender. If someone were suffering from bronchitis you could use pine, eucalyptus or any suitable alternative. Another method of burning essential oils if you do not have the correct tools is to place a couple of drops directly onto a light bulb in a room. This is a very fast and effective way to use oils when you have no other alternative.

Tissues

Alternatively you can place a few drops of essential oils directly onto a tissue or a hankie and inhale directly. This method is an equally effective manner in which to use oils.

Sleeves

A sleeve on a sweater can be used if you need it for emergency purposes. If you are apprehensive about going out and require a confidence booster, just place a couple of Ylang Yang oil directly onto your sleeve and inhale as required. You will be surprised at the outcome.

Specific Guidelines & Cautions for Herbs

Herbs can be used for many purposes such as healing, mood enhancers, for physical, emotional and psychological gains. However, they are extremely potent and can be lethal if not used correctly. Just as you have to be careful with essential oils you must also understand how important it is to adhere to the enclosed recipes. The herbal brews will clearly show you in a step-by-step manner how to measure, mix and make potions for various ailments.

You can grow your own herbs or pick them fresh from nearby woodlands and the strength would be far superior than those bought from the supermarket. Years ago people could just walk through a forestry, down by a stream and identify and pick the herbs they required. Nowadays, the supermarket has come into play and since the industrial revolution, which forced the masses away from the countryside into the towns, thus separating people from Mother nature and the richness of the land. People soon lost their natural ability to go into the wild and pick their own herbs.

With the quickening pace of life, the supermarkets became more and more popular, thus destroying our farming and food cultures. Farmers today are even buying their own food from supermarkets which just goes to show how far away from nature we are getting. Herbs can be used in our foods which can nourish both ourselves and our children. Herbs can dilute fat in items that we intake daily. They are just so many great qualities in fresh herbs that I urge you to try to grow your own. Just follow my guidelines at the end of the book where I will show you how to grow a herbal wheel. This can be grown in a small area in your garden or even in window boxes. Get back to nature and feel the benefits of growing a reaping your own produce.

Ailments
Physical, psychological & spirutual

∿

ANXIETY, STRESS AND OVERWORK
ANGER AND TRANTRUMS
APATHY & LACK OF ATTENTION
APHRODISIAC AND LOVE POTIONS
ABSCESSES, BOILS, ACNE & WOUNDS
ADDICTIONS
ALLERGIES
ARTHRITIS & RHEUMATISM
ASTHMA
BALDNESS
BEREAVEMENT, GRIEF AND SHOCK
BITES, STINGS, BRUISES & CUTS
BRONCHIAL PROBLEMS, FLU COLDS, COUGHS AND CONGESTION
SUNBURN, SKIN PROBLEMS AND BURNS
COLIC, CRAMPS, CONSTIPATION AND INDIGESTION
CIRCULATION
CLAUSTROPHOBIA
CONFIDENCE, COURAGE AND POSITIVE THINKING
CYSTITIS AND URINARY TRACT PROBLEMS
DANDRUFF, DERMATITIS AND ECZEMA
DEPRESSION, MENTAL AND PHYSICAL EXHAUSTION
EARACHE, TINNITUS AND SINUSTIS
FEAR, TERROR, NERVES AND PANIC ATTACKS
GUILT AND HOSTILITY
HYPERTENSION
HYPERACTIVITY
IMMUNE SYSTEM
INSOMNIA
MIGRAINE, HEADACHES AND HANGOVERS
NEURALGIA

OVERWEIGHT
PARANOIA, SELF-CRITICISM AND SHYNESS
PMT & PERIODS
RELAXING AND SELF-ACCEPTANCE
VARICOSE VEINS
WARTS
WORRY

ANXIETY, STRESS AND OVERWORK-
ESSENTIAL OILS

Essential Oils : Bergamont, Neroli, Clary Sage, Marjoram, Lemongrass and Cedarwood.

ANXIETY—Bergamont Oil
STRESS — Cedarwood, Clary Sage and Neroli
OVERWORK PHYSICAL—Clary Sage, Lemongrass, Neroli and Lavender
OVERWORK MENTAL — Clary sage and Neroli.

BERGAMONT: This is an uplifting oil which must never be used for up to three hours before you go out in the sun. Bergamont can never be used for children from the age of 0 up to 12 years old. You can use it in your bath, in a compress or for inhalation.

NEROLI: This is an oil generally used for stress related problems. Overwork, mental stress and shock. It cannot be used for children from the age of 0 up to 12 years old. It can be used restrictively during pregnancy and for people with sensitive skin. You can use this in your bath, as an inhaler or in a compress.

MARJORAM: This oil is classed as a muscle relaxant. It cannot be used for children from the age of 0 up to 12 years old. It is an excellent oil for aches, spasms and sprains. It can be used in your bath, as an inhaler or in a compress.

CLARY SAGE: This is a euphoric oil. It cannot be used for children from the age of 0 up to 12 years old. It must be used restrictively during pregnancy and for people with sensitive skin. It can be used in a bath, as a compress or as an inhaler.

LEMONGRASS: This is a strengthening oil. It cannot be used

for children from the age of 0 up to 12 years old. It must be used restrictively during pregnancy. It is an excellent oil which alleviates nervous exhaustion and muscle aches and pains. It can be used as an insect repellent, a room fragrancer, in your bath or as a compress.

CEDARWOOD: This oil has a composing effect. It cannot be used for children from the age of 0 up to 12 years old. It must be used restrictively during pregnancy. It is a wonderful oil for stress relief, for asthma, bronchitis, dandruff and scattered thinking. You can use this oil in your bath, as an inhaler or as a compress.

ANXIETY, STRESS AND OVERWORK— PROTECTION AMULETS

Herbs: Yarrow, Nettle, Mullein, Snapdragon, Lemon Balm, Rue and Acorn.

INFUSION: Lemon Balm leaves.

STOP ANXIETY OR FEAR: Carry a mixture of nettle and yarrow.

COURAGE: Carry on your person Mullein.

STOP OTHER DECEIVING YOU: Wear a snapdragon.

KEEP ILLNESS AWAY: Wear a sprig of rue around your neck.

REGAIN LOST MANHOOD: Carry an acorn.

ANGER AND TANTRUMS

Essential Oils: Ylang Ylang and Chamomile.

ANGER—Ylang Ylang
TANTRUMS—Chamomile

YLANG YLANG—This oil is for confidence. It cannot be used on children from 0 to 12 years old. This oil is an excellent choice for instilling confidence. It can be used in your bath, as an inhaler or on a compress.

CHAMOMILE—(ROMAN) This oil is for healing and soothing. It can be used by any age group, during pregnancy or on sensitive skin. It is a very diverse oil which can be used for colic, dermatitis, exzema, an overactive mind, trantrums, hot flushes, sensitive skin, swollen joints boils and bed wetting. You can use this oil in your bath, as an inhaler, a compress, massage, as a room fragrancer, on your pillow at night, on a tissue or for scalp treatment.

HERBAL REMEDIES-ANGER AND TANTRUMS

ATTRACT FRIENDLINESS: Wear a heliotope.
NARCISSUS: Promotes peace, scerenity and harmony.
PATCHOULI: A very powerful way to ward off negativity.
CYCLAMEN: Eases anger or tantrums brought on by pain.

APATHY & LACK OF ATTENTION-ESSENTIAL OILS

Essential Oils: Jasmine, Rosemary and Basil.

APATHY- Emotional apathy—Jasmine. Mental or physical apathy—Rosemary.

LACK OF ATTENTION—Basil for short attention span.

JASMINE—This oil is known as an aphrodisiac. It can not be used for children from the age of o to twelve years old. It treats many conditions such as apathy, detatchment, jealousy, sadness, shyness and is an aphrodisiac. This oil can be used in your bath, as an inhaler or on a compress.

ROSEMARY—This oil is known as a stimulant. It cannot be used for children from the age o o to twelve years old. It oil is not suitable for use during pregnancy. This oil can treat a range of ailments such as, short attention span, disorientation, dull memory, bad memory, sluggishness, circulation, constipation, muscle aches and tiredness. You can use this oil in your bath or as an inhaler.

APATHY & LACK OF ATTENTION-HERBS

Herbs: All-spice, Carnations, Eucalyptus, Honeysuckle

ALL SPICE: Anoint daily.

CARNATIONS: For power and energy restoration. Wear when you are tired.

EYCALYPTUS: Recouperation after an illness. Dab on your wrists of forehead.

HONEYSUCKLE: Promotes clarity and quick thinking.

APHRODISIAC, LOVE POTIONS & SPELLS-ESSENTIAL OILS

Essential Oils: Rose Otto, Jasmine , Ylang Ylang and Fragrance of Venus Oil.

FRAGRANGE OF VENUS OIL: This is one of the most potent aphrodisiac oils for women. It cannot be used on children from 0-12 and should only be used by women who really want to attract men. The results of wearing this oil are amazing. It can be used in your bath, as a perfume or an inhaler (see herbs)

ROSE OTTO: This oil is considered cleansing. It cannot be used on children from 0 to 12 years old. Is uses are for weepiness and attachment. It can be used in a bath or as an inhaler.

JASMINE: This oil is consiered an aphrodisiac. It cannot be used on children from 0 to 12 years old. It has many used such as an aphrodisiac, emotional expression, secretive and too introvert or too extrovert. It can be used in your bath, as an inhaler or on a compress.

YLANG YLANG: This oil is considered a confidence booster. It cannot be used on children from 0 to 12 years old. It has many uses such as an aphrodisiac, courage booster and confidence. It can be used in your bath, as an inhaler or on a compress.

APHRODISIAC, LOVE POTIONS & SPELLS-HERBS

Herbs: Lavender, Batchelor's Buttons, Valerian Root, Red Rose, Musk, Bay Leaf, Patchouli, Gardinea, Cinnamon, HenbanE, Orris Root, Rose Petals, Yarrow, Mint, Catnip, Strawberry Leaves, Coltsfoot, Tansy, Vervian and Fragrrance of Venus Oil.

LOVE SACHETS: In order to attract a man, mix together a pinch of Valerian Root, a Bay Leaf, dried Batchelor's Buttons and Lavender. Carry this sachet on your person or sleep with it under your pillow.

LOVE SACHETS: In order to attact a woman, mix together Cinnamon, Henbane and Patchouli. Carry this sachet on your person or sleep with it under your pillow.

LOVE SPELLS: (SACHET) This is one of the most used love spells and an ancient method. It can be made up in a sachet or scattered as follows. Mix up dried Rose Petals, a pinch of Yarrow, a pinch of Catnip, a leaf of Mint, Coltsfoot, Orris Root, Tansy, Strawberry Leaves and a bit of Vervian. This must be mixed only on a Friday night during a full moon. Then you divide the mixture into three parts, the first part you go outside naked and throw up to the Moon. The second part you bring back indoors and scatter it around your bedroom and the third part you make up a sachet with green cloth and wear it on your body.

LOVE CHARMS: Any of these herbs, oils or flowers can be made up into a potion and must not be taken internally; Mandrake, Marjoram, Apple, Aster, Meadowsweet, Batchelor's Buttons, Balm of Gilead, Cumin, Dragon's Blood, Orris Root, Pink Geranium, Rose, Southernwood, Lavender, Loveage, Vrevain, Violet and Yarrow.

FRAGRANGE OF VENUS OIL: If you want to be a completely desirable woman mix together on a Friday Night Jasmine, Red Rose,

Ylang Ylang 2 drops, one drop of Lavender and a bit of musk. You can wear it on your person and watch out.

TO ATTRACT LOVE: Wear a Gardinea.

ADDICTIONS — ESSENTIAL OILS

Essential Oils: Clare Sage & Rose Otto

CLARY SAGE: This oil is known as Euphoric. It cannot be used on children from 0 to 12 years of age. It is not suitable and restricted during pregnancy. It has a number of uses such as addictions, insomnia, claustrophobia, compulsiveness, hostility, depression, obsession, negative thoughts and listlesness. You can use this in your bath and as an inhaler.

ROSE OTTO: This oil is known as a freshening and cleansing oil. It cannot be used on children from 0 to 12 years of age. It has a number of uses which include, love, addictions, hangovers, migraine, allergies, weepy, berevement, regret, self-centeredness and grief. It can be used in a bath or as an inhaler.

ADDICTIONS — HERBS

Herbs & Flowers: Frankincense, Honeysuckle, Hyacinth and Melilot

FRANKINCENSE: Can be worn and is a wonderful oil for purification and blessing.
HONEYSUCKLE: Put a couple of dabs of oil on your temples or carry Honeysuckle as an mind cleanser.
HYACINTH: An oil that can be worn or a small sachet can bring you peace of mind.
MELILOT: Wear this or carry in a sachet to fight depression that addiction can bring.

ABSCESSES, BOILS, ACNE & WOUNDS-ESSENTIAL OILS

Essential Oils: Chamomile, Teatree, Frankincense, and Lavender.

CHAMOMILE: This oil is known for its soothing purposes. Anyone can use it. It is particularly great to relieve the redness of the face associated with Acne. It has many other uses such as the treatment of dermatitis, exzema, tantrums, boils and restlessness. It can be used in your bath, as a compress, dabbed directly onto the area with a cotton bud or for massage.

TEATREE: This oil is an antiseptic. It cannot be used on children from 0 to 12 years old. This oil is particularly useful with regard to clearing up the pimples on your face caused by acne or for the direct treatment onto boils or abscesses. You can use it in your bath or as an inhaler.

FRANKINCENSE:—This oil is a great for rejuvenation. It cannot be used on children form 0 to 12 years old. It is a wonderful oil for weeping abscesses, scarring from acne, cracked and weeping skin, fear, insecurity, nerves, panic attacks and haemorrhoids. It can be used in your bath or as an inhaler.

LAVENDER:—This oil is a great immune system booster. It can be used by all. It is a great oil for treating acne, abscesses, blisters, burns, exhaustion, eczema, insomnia, migraine, nausea, mood swings, irritability, panic attacks and stage fright. You can use it in your bath, as an inhaler, room fragrancer, for massage or diluted can be applied with a cotton bud as an antibiotic.

ABCESSES, BOILS, ACNE & WOUNDS-HERBS

HERBS: Chamomile, dock leaf, garlic, Fenugreek seeds, lavender, St John's Worth and Aloe Vera.

POULTICE: Funugreek seeds.

INFUSION OR TINCTURE: Elder leaves, flowers or berries.

INTERNALLY: Aloe Vera juice.

EXTERNALLY: You can select any of the above and gently use the plants and herbs to rub directly onto the area required.

RAW: Garlic rubbed directly onto the area.

ALLERGIES — ESSENTIAL OILS

Essential Oils: Rose, Melissa or Eucalyptus.

ROSE: This oil is known as a loving and healing oil. It cannot be used on children from 0 to 12 years of age. It has a number of uses which include, allergies,

hayfever, migraine, nerves (worry about the past) and stability. It can be used in your bath, on a compress, for massage or as a room fragrancer.

MELISSA: This oil is Greek for the word bee. It cannot be used on children from 0 to 12 years of age. It has a number of uses which include, heavy periods, allergies and nurturing your female side. It can be used in a bath or as an inhaler.

EUCALYPTUS: This oil is used for your Respitory system. It cannot be used on children from 0 to 12 years of age. It has a number of uses which include, coughs, chestiness, dry cough, jealousy and nosebleeds. It can be used in a bath or as an inhaler.

ALLERGIES — HERBS & FLOWERS

Herbs: Quercitin, Nettles, Natureade Spray, Decongest Herbal, Enchinacea and Green Tea.

QUERCITIN: Is made up from grape seeds or green tea. It can reduced the effect of the allergy by calming swollen membranes.

NETTLES: Are a wonderful way of reducing itchy patches or redness associates with allergies. They focus on the sinuses and mucous menbras.

DECONGEST HERBAL: This can also be bought on the internet and is a wonderful way of reducing allergies, bacterial infections and viral infections. This product is not suitable for children. It is not suitable for that are sensive to caffeine, have kidney, heart problems or hypertension.

GREEN TEA: This oriental tea has strong antioxidants and is an antibacterial. It can be taken up to 3 or 4 times daily.

ENCHINECEA: This is to build up a run down immune system.

ARTHRITIS AND RHEUMATISM-
ESSENTIAL OILS

E ssential Oils: Chamomile, Lavender and Juniper.

CHAMOMILE: (ROMAN) This oil is known to sooth. It can be used by anyone. It is used particularly for redness caused by arthritis. It can be used in your bath, on a compress or for massage.

JUNIPER: This oil is known to alleviate toxins in your system. It cannot be used by children from 0 to 12 years of age. It should not be used during pregnancy and if so only very restrictively. This oil is used on the swelling associated with arthritis and can be used in your bath, on a compress or for massage.

LAVENDER: This oil is excellent for your immune system. It can be used by any age. It is particularly useful for pain associated with arthritis and can be used as a compress, in your bath, as an inhaler, directly onto the site, for massage, on sensitive skin and as a room fragrancer.

ᕫ

ARTHRITIS & RHEUMATISM—HERBS

Herbs: Ginger Root, Valerian, Comfrey, Arnica oil or cream and Devil's Claw.

DEVIL'S CLAW: 1 to three grams of powder in a capsule.
GINGER ROOT: This herb is known for alleviating joint discomfort and promoting joint health. Ginger is a wonderful herb for the symtoms of arthritis.
VALERIAN: This herb is used for purification.

ARNICA: Cream or oil to be rubbed directly into the area.

COMFREY: This herb is used for protection and rebuilding the immune system.

ASTHMA — ESSENTIAL OILS

Essential Oils: Eucalyptus, Cedarwood and Cypress.

EUCALYPTUS: This oil is known for cleansing and clearing of the respitory system. It cannot be used by children from the age of 0 to 12 years of age. It is not recommended for use if receiving homoepathic treatment. This oil is sometimes used as a chest rub and is a wonderful for treating asthma, bronchitis, colds, headaches, catarrh, sinusitis or congestion. It can be used in your bath or as a room fragrancer.

CEDARWOOD: This oil is known for its composing qualities. It cannot be used for children from 0 to 12 years of age. It must be used restrictively during pregnancy. This is a wonderful for asthma, bronchitis or scattered thoughts. It can be used in your bath, an inhaler or on a compress.

CYPRESS: This oil is known as an astringent. It cannot be used for children from the age of 0 to 12 years old. It has many qualities and is wonderful for the treatment of asthma, coughs, dry cough and nosebleeds. It can be used in your bath or as an inhaler.

ASTHMA — HERBS

HERBS — Citrus Peel, Sage, Ginger, Roman Chamomile Flowers, Gumplant leaves and flowers.

SAGE LEAVES: Burn and inhale.
CITRUS PEEL: You can use either the peel or an orange, lemon or any citrus fruit. Use fresh and inhale to dicongest your respiratory system.

GUMPLANT LEAVES & FLOWERS: 500 ML Infusion—5ml per day.

GINGER ROOT: This herb is known for alleviaging discomfort for both respiratory and joint discomfort.

ROMAN CHAMOMILE FLOWERS: Infusion as per Gumplant Leaves & Flowers.

BALDNESS — ESSENTIAL OILS

Essential oils: Thyme, Rosemary, Cedarwood and Lavender.

(Use a base oil (almond oil) and pour in two drops of each the above essential oils. Massage into your scalp daily)

These oils cannot be used for children from the age of 0 to 12 years of age. It is not recommended to use during pregnancy. The mixture of the four oils above can be massaged daily into your scalp to prevent baldness and reverse hair loss.

THYME: This is an anti-bacterial oil. It cannot be used for children from the age of 0 to 12 years of age and is not recommended during pregnancy. It can be mixed with the above oils to treat baldness and is also excellent for throat infections.

ROSEMARY: This oil is known as a stimulant. It cannot be used for children from the age of 0 to 12 years of age and it is not recommended during pregnancy. Rosemary has many uses such as, baldness, chilblaines, circulation, exercise, dull memory, disorientation, indecisiveness and tiredness. Mix with the other three oils and massage onto scalp.

CEDARWOOD: This oil is know for its composing qualities. It cannot be used for children from 0 to 12 years of age. It must be used restrictively during pregnancy. This oil can be mixed with above oils and massaged into the scalp.

LAVENDER: This oil is excellent to reboost your immune system. It can be used by all. It treats many conditions such as baldness, bedwetting, bruises, burns, insomnia, impatience, paranoia, relaxation and panic attacks. Mix with the three other oils above and massage directly onto your scalp.

ॐ

BALDNESS — HERBS

Herbs: Don Quai

DON QUAI: This contains over 12 natural herbs and can be bought online from CHINESETREATMENTS.COM

BIZZARE TREATMENTS: Pure unrefined Pennysylvania crude oil — rub into your scalp daily.

BEREAVEMENT, GRIEF AND SHOCK-ESSENTIAL OILS

Essential Oils: Melissa, Neroli, Frankincense, Hyssop and Rose.

MELISSA: This oil is known for its female side. It cannot be used on children from 0 to 12 years old. If you are in an extreme state of shock you should mix this oil with Neroli. This oil is a wonderful oil for shock, heavy periods and your feminine side. It can be used in your bath or as an inhaler.

NEROLI: This oil is known as a stress reliever. It cannot be used for children from 0 to 12 years old. As above, if you are in a dreadful state of shock mix this oil with Melissa. Other wonderful attributes include, broken veins, hysteria, shock, stress and exhaustion. It can be used in your bath.

FRANKINCENSE: This oil is known for rejuvenating. It cannot be used on children from 0 to 12 years old. This oil is excellent if you have suffered a recent bereavement, have prolonged grief, fear, insecurity, panic attacks, self criticism or are undisciplined. You can use this oil in your bath or as an inhaler.

HYSSOP: This is known as a stabilising oil. It cannot be used on children from 0 to 12 years. It cannot be used on people who suffer with epilepsy or if you are pregnant. Hyssop is an extremely potent oil and must be used sparingly. It is an excellent oil for grief and hypertension. It can be used in your bath, as an inhaler or on a compress.

❧

BEREAVEMENT, GRIEF AND SHOCK-HERBS

HERBS & FLOWERS: Basil, Bay Laurel, Dill, Fennell, Mistletoe, Rosemary, Snapdragon.

(SACHET): White cotton cloth about 6inches square, red thread.

TO MAKE UP THIS SACHET: Mix together a small amount of all of the above herbs in an earthenware bowl. Spread your cloth down on a table and transfer the herbs to the centre of the cloth. Gathering up the corners of the cloth draw them together and tightly bind with the red thread. Tie twelve knots in the thread and carry your sachet on your person. If you wish to make this up without a sachet simply gather all seven herbs by the stems, hang upside down and put them in whichever room you require.

BITES, STINGS, BRUISES & CUTS- ESSENTIAL OILS

Essential Oils: Lavender, Teatree.

LAVENDER: This oil is known to boost your natural immune system. It can be used by anyone. It is one of the most used and popular oils and is used for the treatment of bites, stings, absesses, acne, blisters, restlessness, stagefright, dermatitis, earache, exezema, overwork and worry. It can be used in your bath, as an inhaler, on a compress, on a cotton bud and placed directly over the area, massage, room fragrancer, on sensitive skin, a few drops on a tissue or your pillow.

TEATREE: This oil is known as an antiseptic. It cannot be used on children from 0 to age 12. It has many uses which include cuts, acne, thrush, candida & acne.

It can be used in your bath or as an inhaler. For particularly bad bites or stings you can apply (diluted) on the area in question.

BITES AND STINGS — HERBS

Herbs & Flowers: Dock leaf and lavender.

DOCK LEAF: This ancient method is known by most people today. If you get a sting you rub the dock leaf directly onto the area.

LAVENDER: Fresh lavender can also be used as a dock leaf. Rub the fresh lavender directly onto the area required.

BRONCHIAL, FLU, COUGHS & CONGESTION-ESSENTIAL OILS

There are so many types of flu, colds, coughs—I have had to be very specific with these ailments.

Essential Oils; Cedarwood, Cypress, Pine, Sandalwood, Eucalyptus, Cinnamon and Black Pepper.

BRONCHITIS: (CEDARWOOD & PINE)—(mixed)—ALL can use in a bath, massage or as an inhaler.

COUGH: (CYPRESS)—Children from 0-12 cannot use. It can be used in your bath or as an inhaler.

CATARRH: (SANDALWOOD)—Children from 0-12 cannot use. It can be used in your bath, as in inhaler or on a compress.

CONGESTION: (EUCALYPTUS)—Children from 0-12, or people using homoeopathic treatment cannot use. Can be used in your bath, as an inhaler.

FLU: (CINNAMON)—Children from 0-12, pregnant women or those with sensitive skin cannot use this oil. It can be used in your bath, inhaler or compress.

FLU: (BLACK PEPPER)—Children from 0-12 or people using homoeopathic treatment cannot use. It can be used in your bath, as an inhaler or compress.

BRONCHIAL, FLU, COUGHS & CONGESTION—HERBS

Herbs: Green tea, Pine, Cearwood, Mint, Anise Seed, Coltsfoot flowers & leaves and Garlic

All of the above herbs are highly useful in treating bronchitis, flu, coughs and congestion. It is really a question of selecting your particular favourite.

INTERNALLY: Anise seed and Garlic. This can be taken as a syrup, tincture or an infusion. Garlic can be eaten raw.

SUNBURN, SKIN PROBLEMS & BURNS-
ESSENTIAL OILS

There are so many different types of skin problems I have to be very specific in this section.

Essential Oils: Geranium, Neroli, Lavender, Sandalwood, Frankincense, Patchouli and Chamomile.

SUNBURN: (LAVENDER)-Boosts your immune system, can be used by all. Use in a bath, a compress or mild massage.

BURNS: (LAVENDER & CHAMOMILE)-Sooths and heals. Can be used by all. Use in a cool bath or on a compress.

SKIN PROBLEMS: (GERANIUM, NEROLI, LAVENDER, SANDALWOOD AND CHAMOMILE)

Inflamed Skin: Chamomile to sooth. Can be used by all. You can put it in your bath or on a compress.

Blotches: Geranium for balancing. Cannot be used by children from 0-12 years. Can be used in your bath.

Chapped: Sandalwood for expression. Cannot be used by children from 0-12 years. Can be used in your bath, inhaler or on a compress.

Weeping Eczema: Lavender. Can be used by all. Use in a bath or on a compress.

Broken Veins: Neroli for skin stress relief. Cannot be used by children from 0-12 years. Use in your bath.

Cracked: Patchouli heals cracked skin. It cannot be used by children from 0-12 years. Use in your bath.

Dry: Geranium & sandalwood for balancing the skin. Cannot be used by children from 0-12 years. Use in your bath or for massage.

Itchy: Lavender. This oil can be used by all. It can be used in your bath, as a compress or for massage.

◈

SUNBURN, SKIN PROBLEMS & BURNS-HERBS

Herbs: Caldndula Oil and Aloe Juice.

SUNBURN: Externally rub with Calendula Oil or Aloe Juice.
BURNS: Externally rub with Aloe Juice.
SKIN PROBLEMS: Externally apply Aloe Juice.

COLIC, CRAMPS, CONSTIPATION AND INDEGESTION -OILS

Essential Oils: Chamomile, Cardamon,Fennell, Rosemary & Black Pepper.

CHAMOMILE: (ROMAN) This is a soothing oil and can be used by all. It is a wonderful oil for colic, nettle rash, sensitive and inflamed skin, sprains, overactive mind and worry. It can be used in your bath, as an inhaler, for massage, as a room fragrance or a few drops on your pillow.

CARDAMON: This oil is an expansive oil. It cannot be used for children from 0-12 years old. It is a great remedy for colic or any digestive problems, confusion or selfishness. It can be used in your bath, as an inhaler or on a compress.

FENNELL: This is a normalising oil. It cannot be used for children from 0-12 years old or during pregnancy. It can be used for bloated abodomens, colic, cellulitis, flatulence, or overweight. It can be used in a bath or as an inhaler.

ROSEMARY: This oil is known as a stimulant. It cannot be used for children from 0-12 years or during pregnancy. It is a wonderful oil for constipation, muscle ache, tendons and disorientation. You can use it in your bath or as an inhaler.

BLACK PEPPER: This oil is known for its penetration qualities. It cannot be used on children from 0-12 years and is not suitable if you are receiving homoeopathic treatment. This is a great oil for constipation, fever, stomach pains, cramps and indegestion. It can be used in your bath, as an inhaler or on a compress.

COLIC, CRAMPS, CONSTIPATION & INDESGESTION- HERBS

Herbs or Flowers—Elder leaves, flowers or berries, thyme leaves, cloves, pepperment & ginger.

EXTERNALLY: Use thyme leaves for inhalation.

INTERNALLY: Eat elder leaves, flower or berries in a very small amount as an infusion.

INTERNALLY: Mix Cloves, Peppermint and ginger and take as an infusion. Either one or these herbs will do on their own or you can combine three.

CIRCULATION — ESSENTIAL OILS

Essential Oils — Rosemary

ROSEMARY: This is known as a stimulant. It cannot be used for children from 0-12 years or during pregnancy. This oil is a wonderful oil for circulation problems, exercise, hangover, leathargy, mental stimulation and sluggishness. It can be used in your bath or as an inhaler.

CIRCULATION — HERBS

HERBS — Rosemary

EXTERNALLY — Can be burnt on a fire as a room fragrancer or an inhaler.

CLAUSTROPHOBIA-ESSENTIAL OILS

Essential Oils — Clary Sage and Frankincense

CLARY SAGE: This oil is known as Euphoric. It cannot be used for children from 0-12 years, during pregnancy or on sensitive skin types. It is a great oil for claustrophobia, addictions, depression, recurrent dreams, negative thoughts, over-analytical mind and insomnia. It can be used in your bath, as an inhaler or on a compress.

FRANKINCENSE: This is known as a rejuvenating oil. It cannot be used on children from 0-12 years. It is a great oil for claustrophobia, fear, nerves, panic attacks, self criticism, acne scarring and weeping abscesses. It can be used in your bath or as an inhaler.

CLAUSTROPHIBIA-HERBS

Herbs: Frankincense.

FRANKINCENSE: As above you can burn Frankincense as a room fragrancer or an inhaler.

CONFIDENCE, COURAGE AND POSITIVE THINKING-OILS

Essential Oils: Jasmine, Frankincense and Lavender.

JASMINE: This oil is known as an aphrosisiac. It cannot be used on children from the age of 0-12 years. It is a wonderfully uplifting oil and can treat confidence, fear, apathy, detatchment, rigidity and stress. It can be used in your bath, as an inhaler or on a compress.

FRANKINCENSE: This oil is known as a rejuvenating oil. It cannot be used on children from 0-12 years. It is very effective on working on nerves, fear, panic attacks and is a great conficence booster. It can be used in your bath (mixed with Jasmine), as an inhaler or on a compress.

LAVENDER: Healing oil that can be used by everyone. It works very effectively on relaxing your nerves, hysteria, fear of people, fright, insomnia, irrationality, negative thoughts, panic attacks, stage fright as well as dermatitis, earache, eczema cracked and weeping, nosebleeds, PMT, pregnancy and burns.

CONFIDENCE, COURAGE AND POSITIVE THINKING-HERBS

Herbs: Oats and St John's Worth.

INTERNALLY: As a infusion or a tincture. Oats or St John's Worth flowers can be used as an uplifting and confidence giving remedy.

CYSTITUS, URINARY TRACT PROBLEMS-
ESSENTIAL OILS

Essential Oils:- Juniper and Sandalwood.

JUNIPER: This oil is known for toxic elimination from the body. It cannot be used on children from 0-12 years or during pregnancy. It is a wonderful oil for cystitus, burning associates with cystitus, cramps, scanty periods and lethargy. It can be used in your bath or as a compress.

❧

CYSTITUS, URINARY TRACT PROBLEMS-
HERBS

Herbs: Birch Leaves, Enchinacea root, Enchinacea leaves, Aloe.

INTERNALLY: As an infusion or a tincture. Mix up three of the above herbs or flowers and use to combat the burning sensation and cramps associated with cystitus or any urinary tract problems.

DANDRUFF, DERMATITIS AND ECZEMA-ESSENTIAL OILS

There are so many different mixtures and skin disorders that I have had to be very specific on the mixture of essential oils.

ESSENTIAL OILS: Cypress and Cedarwood-scalp treatment.

DERMATITIS: Mix up Rosemary, Geranium, Lavender and Chamomile.

ECZEMA: WEEPING—Mix up Lavender Frankincense.

ECZEMA: SENSITIVE—Mix up Lavender and Geranium.

ECZEMA: BURNING- Apply Chamomile.

ECZEMA: ITCHY—Apply Chamomile.

As outlined in all the oils above Lavender and Chamomile can be used by all in a bath, for gentle massage or on a compress. Cypress, Cedarwood, Rosemary, Geranium and Frankincense are not suitable for children from the age 0-12 years old and not during pregnancy. Check if you have sensitive skin before use.

DANDRUFF, DERMATITIS AND ECZEMA-HERBS

EXZEMA AND DERMATITIS: Herb required to use externally as an ointment, a paste or a poultice is Comfrey.

DANDRUFF: MINT—Prepare as an ointment or a tincture and apply directly onto the scalp.

DEPRESSION, MENTAL & PHYSICAL EXHAUSTION—OILS

E ssential Oils—Bergamont, Clary Sage and Rosemary.

BERGAMONT: This oil is known for its uplifting qualities. It cannot be used on children from the ages of 0-12 years, never use for about three hours before you go out into the direct sunlight as it may cause pigmentation problems. This is one of the most valuable oils for fighting depression and mental or physical exhaustion.

It treats many ailments such as depression, anxiety, PMT, negative thinking, regret, stress and shyness. It can be used in your bath, as an inhaler or on a compress.

CLARY SAGE: This oil is known for its euphoric qualities. It cannot be used on children from 0-12 years or never during pregnancy. It has many qualities which fight against exhausion, addiction, insomnia, obsession, hostility, depression and stress. It can be used in your bath or as an inhaler.

ROSEMARY: This oil is known as a stimulant. It cannot be used for children from 0-12 years of age or during pregnancy. It is a wonderful oil for clarity, lethargy, bad memory, circulation, migraine, the blues or sluggishness. It can be used in your bath or as an inhaler.

DEPRESSION, MENTAL & PHSICAL EXHAUSION-HERBS

Herbs—Oats and St John's Worth flowers.

INTERNALLY: Use as an infusion or a tincture.

EARACHE, TINNITUS AND SINUSTIS-
ESSENTIAL OILS

Essential Oils: Lavender, Eucalyptus, Peppermint.

LAVENDER: This oil can be used by all. It is a wonderful if mixed with Eucalyptus for dealing with head pain associated with Sinustis. If you mix this with Peppermint is can treat Tinnitus or alone it can assist with earaches. It can be used as a compress, an inhaler or in your bath.

EUCALYPTUS: This oil is known as a soother for your respitory system. It cannot be used by children from 0-12 years of age. It can be mixed with lavender to assist with pain associates with tinnitus. It can be used in your bath.

PEPPERMINT: This oil is known as a cooling oil. It cannot be used by children from 0-12 years of age. It is a wonderful mental stimulant, assists in aches and pains, for headaches, studying, tinnitus nausea or sensitivity to movement. It can be used in your bath or as an inhaler.

EARACHE, TINNITUS AND SINUSTIS-
HERBS

Herbs: Goldenseal capsules, enchinacea.

EARACHE: INTERNALLY—as a tincture or infusion you can use Goldenseal capsules.
SINUSTIS: EXTERNALLY—Enchinacea can be used as a rub on the sinus.
TINNITUS: EXTERNALLY—Enchinacea can be used as a rub for tinnitus.

FEAR, TERROR, NERVES & PANIC ATTACKS-ESSENTIAL OILS

This section has so many aspects I have had to break them down individually.

FEAR OF FAILURE—Lavender & Sandalwood mixed. In a bath, as a inhler, room fragranger or tissue. Not suitable for children from 0-12 years.

TERROR: Frankincense & Rose mixed. In you bath, as an inhaler, room fragrancer, massage. Not suitable for children 0-12 or during pregnancy.

FRIGHT: Frankincense & Lavender mixed. In your bath, as an inhaler, room fragrancer or massage. Not suitable for children 0-12 or pregnancy.

OF PEOPLE: Lavender & Ylang Ylang mixed. In your bath, as an inhaler, room fragrancer or massage. Not suitable for children 0-12 years.

PANIC ATTACKS: Frankincense & Lavender mixed. In your bath, as an inhaler, room fragrancer, massage. Not suitable for children 0-12 or pregnancy.

NERVES: Camphor, Melissa & Sandalwood mixed. In your bath, inhaler, room fragrancer, massage. Not suitable for children 0-12 or pregnancy.

STAGEFRIGHT: Lavender & Ylang Ylang. In your bath, inhaler, room fragrancer, massage or tissue. Not suitable for children 0-12 or pregnancy.

INSECURITY: Lavender, Sandalwood & Frankincense. In your bath, inhaler, room fragrancer or massage. Not suitable for children 0-12 or pregnancy.

FAINTING: Rosemary & Basil. Can be used as an inhaler. Not suitable for children from 0-12 or during pregnancy.

NAUSEA: Lavender. Can be used by all in your bath, as an inhaler, as a room fragrancer or for massage.

FEAR, TERROR, NERVES & PANIC ATTACKS — HERBS

NAUSEA: Internally as an infusion. Cloves, peppermint and Ginger.

PANIC ATTACKS: Lavender. Can be used as an inhaler, room fragrance or under your pillow.

GUILT AND HOSTILITY- ESSENTIAL OILS

Essential Oils: Ylang Ylang, Clary Sage, Marjoram.

YLANG YLANG: This oil is known as a confidence booster. It cannot be used by children from the age of 0-12 or during pregnancy. It is an excellent oil for many psychological conditions such as guilt, hostility, irritability, panic attacks, shyness and self esteem. It can be used in a bath, as an inhaler or on a compress.

CLARY SAGE: Mix Clary Sage, Marjoram and Ylang Ylang for hostility. It cannot by used by children from the age of 0-12 or during pregnancy. It is an excellent mix for hostility and can be used in your bath, as an inhaler, for massage or as a room fragrancer.

MARJORAM: This oil is known for muscle relaxant qualities. It cannot be used by children from 0-12 years or during pregnancy. It has many qualities and can be used for hostility, irrational thoughts, muscle relaxant, mental strain and overwork. It can be used in your bath, as an inhaler or on a compress

❧

GUILT AND HOSTILITY-HERBS

MARJORAM: Can be used as an infusion. Mix up a little marjoram and follow the guidelines for making an infusion. This cannot be used by children from the age of 0-12 or during pregnancy.

HYPERTENSION — ESSENTIAL OILS

Essential Oils: Hyssop

HYSSOP: This oil is know as a stabaliser. It must be used in very small amounts and is not suitable for children from the age of 0-12, people who suffer from epilepsy or during pregnancy. It can be used in your bath, as an inhaler or on a compress.

HYPERTENSION — HERBS

HERBS: Thyme

EXTERNALLY: Burn Thyme and inhale.

HYPERACTIVITY- ESSENTIAL OILS

Essential Oils: Clary Sage, Marjoram and Lavender.

To combat hyperactivity you need to mix all three oils above. These oils cannot be used on children from the age of 0-12 years or during pregnancy. The oils can be used in your bath, as an inhaler, room fragrancer or for massage.

HYPERACTIVITY-HERBS

Herbs: Oats

OATS: INTERNALLY—As a tincture or infusion.

IMMUNE SYSTEM—ESSENTIAL OILS

Essential Oils for stimulating the Immune System—Lavender

LAVENDER: This is the most used and well known essential oil. It can be used by all and is excellent in treating the immune system. Other ailments that this oil treats include cuts, dermatitis, earache, exhaustion, insomnia, overwork, nerves, relaxation, restless mind, burns, sprains and panic attacks. It can be used in your bath, as an inhaler, for massage, as a compress or as a room fragrancer.

IMMUNE SYSTEM—HERBS

HERBS—ENCHINACEA

ENCHINACEA: INTERNALLY—This is a wonderful herb for totally revitalising and boosting your immune system. It can be used as an infusion or as a tincture.

INSOMNIA—ESSENTIAL OILS

E ssential Oils: Clary Sage and Lavender.

Mix both of the above oils together for insomnia. These oils cannot be used for children from the age of 0-12 years. They can be mixed and put into your bath, used as an inhaler, on a compress, put a couple of drops on your pillow or for gentle massage.

INSOMNIA—HERBS

HERBS: Hops, Passion Flower and Valerian.

INTERNALLY: The three herbs above can be mixed together and used as an tincture or an infusion for insomnia. This is an excellent way to get a good night's sleep. Take about 30 minutes before bedtime.

MIGRAINE, HEADACHES AND HANGOVERS-ESSENTIAL OILS

This is another area where I must be very specific due to the many kinds of ailments

HEADACHE WITH A COLD: Eucalyptus Oil is the best oil to alleviate a headache with a cold. It cannot be used by children from 0-12 or during pregnancy. It can be used in your bath, for massage, as an inhaler, room fragrancer or on a compress.

HEADACHE TENSION: Lavender. This oil can be used by all. For a tension headache simply put lavender drops in your bath, as a room fragrancer, on your pillow, as an inhaler or on a compress applied to your head.

HEADACHE MIGRAINE: Lavender. Apply as above. When a migrane has settled you can also apply Rosemary to your temples.

HEADACHE SINUS: Basil. This is a clearing oil and cannot be used by children from the age of 0-12, during pregnancy or on sensitive skintypes. It can be used in your bath, as an inhaler or on a compress.

HANGOVER: Rose and Juniper mixed. This cannot be used by children from the age 0-12 or during pregnancy. It can be used in your bath, as an inhaler, on a compress or gently massaged into your temples.

℘

MIGRAINE, HEADACHES AND HANGOVERS-HERBS

Herbs: Thyme and Lavender

THYME: Thyme can be burned and be inhaled to alleviate migraine, headaches and hangover.

LAVENDER: Fresh Lavender can be placed in a sachet under your pillow or inhaled.

NEURALGIA — Essential Oils

E ssential Oils: Peppermint

PEPPERMINT: This oil is known for its cooling qualities. It cannot be used on children from the age 0-12 years. This oil is used for many purposes such as neuralgia, studying, migraine, nausea and tinnitus nausea. It can be used in your bath or as an inhaler.

NEURALGIA-HERBS

Herbs: St John's Worth and fresh lemon.

INTERNALLY: St John's Worth can be used internally to alleviate neuralgia.

EXTERNALLY: Rub the skin of a fresh Lemon over the area and this will alleviate neuralgia.

OVERWEIGHT—ESSENTIAL OILS

E ssential Oils: Patchoili and Fennell.

PATCHOILI: This oil is known for it's pensive qualities. It cannot be used on children from 0-12 years old. It can be used for overweight, apprehension and clarity. It can be used in your bath or as an inhaler.

FENNELL: This oil is known for it's normalising qualities. It cannot be used on children from 0-12 years old or during pregnancy. Fennell can be used for treating overweight, excessive appetite, cellulitis, indigestion and nausea from overeating. It can be used alone or mixed with Patchouli and used in your bath or as an inhaler.

OVERWEIGHT—HERBS

Herbs: Cloves, Peppermint and Ginger.

A mixture of the three herbs above can be used internally as an infusion to treat overweight or excessive appetite.

PARANOIA, SELF-CRITICISM AND SHYNESS-ESSENITAL OILS

S ELF CRITICISM: Ylang Ylang, Frankincense and Sandalwood.
PARANOIA: Rosewood, Lavender and Frankincense.
SHYNESS: Ylang Ylang, Bergamont and Jasmine.

These oils can be used as above—three mixed together. They cannot be used on children from 0-12 years, during pregnancy or directly onto sensitive skin types. They can be used in your bath, as an inhaler, on a compress, as a room fragrancer or for massage.

᪥

PARANOIA, SELF-CRITICISM AND SHYNESS—HERBS

Herbs: Valerian and Spearmint.

VALERIAN: Peacefulness and scerenity. Valerian can be used as a tincture or as an infusion.
SPEARMINT: For healing. Spearmint can be used as a tincture or as an infusion.

PMT AND PERIODS — ESSENTIAL OILS

As there are many varieties of problems associates with PMT and Periods I have had to be very specific in this section

IRREGULAR PERIODS: Cypress. This cannot be used by children from 0-12 years and can be used in your bath or as a massage oil.

HEAVY PERIODS: Melissa and Gerarium. This cannot be used by children from 0-12 years. This mix can be used in your bath or for massage.

SCANTY PERIODS: Juniper. This cannot be used on children from 0-12 years. It can be used in your bath or for massage.

PMT:

MOOD SWINGS: Geranium. This cannot be used by children from 0-12 years. It can be used in your bath or for massage

DEPRESSION: Bergamont. This cannot be used by children from 0-12 years. It can be used in your bath or for massage.

WATER RETENTION: Juniper. This cannot be used by children from 0-12 years. It can be used in your bath or for massage.

IRRITABILITY: Lavender. This can be used by all. It can be used in a bath, for massage, inhalation and room fragrancer.

WEEPING: Rose. This cannot be used by children form 0-12 years. It can be used in your bath or for massage.

PMT AND PERIODS — HERBS

Herbs — Evening Primrose Oil, Lady's Mantle, Hops and Black Cohosh.

INTERNALLY: Evening primrose oil.

INTERNALLY FOR HEAVY PERIODS: Lady's Mantle can be used as a tinture or an infusion.

EXTERNALLY: For pain relief Valerian, hops or Black Cohosh.

RELAXING AND SELF-ACCEPTANCE-ESSENTIAL OILS

Essential Oils: Lavender, Marjoram, Rosewood, Clary Sage and Ginger.

RELAXING: Mix Lavender, Marjoran, Rosewood and Clary Sage. This cannot be used by children from 0-12 years or during pregnancy. It can be used in your bath, as an inhaler or for gentle massage.

SELF-ACCEPTANCE: Ginger. This is known as a digestion oil. It cannot be used on children from 0-12 years old or on sensitive skin types. It is a wonderful psychological oil for self-acceptance and it also treats cold symptoms and arthritis. It can be used in your bath, as an inhaler or on a compress.

RELAXING AND SELF-ACCEPTANCE — HERBS

Herbs: Valerian, Oats, St John's Worth.

INTERNALLY: Valerian, St John's Worth and Oats. Any of these three will alleviate stress and promote self-acceptance. They can be used internally as a tincture, in tablet form or as an infusion.

VARICOSE VEINS — ESSENTIAL OILS

E ssential Oils: Lavender and Cypress.

Both of these oils can be mixed together to treat varicose veins. This treatment may take a little time and cannot be used on children from 0-12 years or during pregnancy. This mixture can be used in your bath or as a compress directly onto the veins.

VARICOSE VEINS — HERBS

INTERNALLY: Horse Chestnut can be used internally as a tincture.

EXTERNALLY: Calendula and witch hazel can be used externally as a compress to treat varicose veins.

WARTS — ESSENTIAL OILS

Essential Oils: Lemon

LEMON: This is known as a refreshing oil. It cannot be used on children from the age of 0-12 years. It can be used directly onto the wart with the aid of a cotton bud or on a small compress.

WARTS — HERBS

INTERNALLY: Thuja can be used internally as a tincture to treat warts.

EXTERNALLY: Garlic or dandelion juice. Either of these can be used directly onto the wart and applied several times a day.

WORRY—ESSENTIAL OILS

Essential Oils: Lavender and Chamomile.

LAVENDER: This is the most used of all oils and can be used by all. It can be used in your bath, as an inhaler, a room fragrancer, for massage and on your pillow. It treats so many different kinds of physical and psychological conditions such as abscesses, acne, worry, fear, negative thoughts, nerves, migraine, nausea and many more.

CHAMOMILE: (ROMAN)—Is known as a soothing oil. It can be used by all. It treats many ailments such as worry, overactive or restless mind, tantrums, hot flushes, sensitive skin, swollen joints. It can be used in your bath, as an inhaler, as a room fragrancer, for massage and can be mixed with Lavender to increase the strength.

WORRY—HERBS

Herbs: Oats, Hops and Valerian.

EXTERNALLY: Hops can be used externally on a compress.
INTERNALLY: Oats or Valerian. This can be used as an infusion, a tincture or in tablet form.

Wands, Ancient Secret Potions and Supersticions
How to make a Wand

You will need a magic knife of which there are two types. Firstly, you have the athame and secondly the magic knife. The athame is used for energy purposes and for symbolic rituals whereas the magic knife is used for banishing, exorcising, cutting herbs, cloth and for enchantments. There are many various kind of wands made up of various woods so you can select one or make them all.

To make a knife you must select one with a wooden handle and a metal blade. It must then be wrapped in a white linen cloth and hidden until the arrival of the next full moon. At sunset, go to your hidden place, somewhere where you will not be disturbed. If you could go to a forest nearby a clear running stream this would be ideal. Light a fire made of old wood. You will also need fresh spring water if there is no stream available as this rite can be done within the confines of your own garden.

The next stage is to bury your knife in the earth up as far as the hilt and kneel before it. Place both of your hands on either side of the knife and face North and say;

'*I conjure thee o knife of steel, by the powers of all the earth, that thou shall be of service to me in my art*'. With your hand that you normally use for writing you then pull the blade from the earth. Move to the highest spot available and hold your knife up to the sky, face East and say; '*I conjure thee of knife of steel, by all the powers of the winds, that thou shall be of service to me in my art*'. Return back to the flames of the fire and place the blade within the flames say; '*I conjure thee o knife of steel, by the powers of all fires and flames, that thou shalt be of service to me in my art*'. Finally, bring yout knife to the stream (or in natural spring water), face west and say; '*I conjure thee of knife of steel, by all the powers within water, that thou shall be of service to me in my art'.* Now wrap your knife in a clean white cloth, pour water from the stream over it and return home. Always remember to keep your knife sharp at all times.

Types of Wand

To make your wand you must do so during a waxing moon at night. All wands must be made of freshly cut wood from a living tree. Here are some of the types of wands you can make and the specific purpose for each one;

WAND OF PROSPERITY: Must be made from a branch of a Fir tree.

WAND FOR LOVE: Must be made from a branch of an Apple tree.

WAND FOR HEALING: Must be made from a branch of an Ash tree.

WAND FOR PURIFICATION: Must be made from a branch of a Birch tree.

WAND FOR EXORCISMS: Must be made from a branch of a Elder tree.

WAND FOR PROTECTION: Must be made from a branch of a Rowan tree.

WAND FOR MAGIC: Must be made from a branch of a Willow tree.

When you are going to cut your particular branch that you require, you firstly bathe, dress in clean cloths, go up to the tree, circle it three times clockwise and pointing your knife towards the tree, say; *'O mighty and strong tree I beseech you to offer me some of your wood to construct a wand which will aid me in the process of my art. You are strong and great as I ask this of you o great tree'.* Then select a branch that looks straight and no more than 30 inches in length. Remember you have to shape your wand and sand it down and it cannot be more than half an inch in width.

With your magic knife cut the piece from the tree gently. Thank the tree by tieing a red ribbon in the shape of a bow around the trunk or bury an offering such as a precious stone at the base of the tree.

When you bring the piece of wood back to your home you then remove any growth, knarls and sand it down removing all of the bark. Do this until your piece of wood is shiny. Take a clean cloth and pour frankincense or sandlewood oil onto it and rub into your wand. Wrap your wand in a yellow clean cloth and put in a dark place for seven days and seven nights. On the seventh night take out your wand and lay it down on fresh earth. Finally, you touch your wand with the blade of your magic knife and say; *'O wand of (willow, apple, ash, rowan, birch, fir or elder), whichever type it may be, I consecrate thee by the virtues of the water, earth, fire and air. I wish thou to be possessed of powers and magic that aid me in my art'.*

Holding you wand in your strong hand and pointed upwards, invoke to the god that you worship and repeat the above incantation facing North, South, East and West. Finally, call on the powers of earth, fire, wind and water to bless your wand.

Divination & Clairvoyance

This ancient formula is used today by modern day witches, psychics, clairvoyants, crystal ball seers, meditation and tarot card readers.

'You burn the following mixture to strengthen your inner sight; Juniper, Patchouli, Sandalwood and Gum Mastic'.

Take equal parts of the above powered herbs, mix well and slightly wet them with a few drops of Ambergis oil or Musk. If you canot locate the above oils you can use Nutmeg and Clove. Let the mixture stand for one night, place it into a jar or container, leave the lid sightly open. This mixture must be done on a Wednesday night.

Wind Listening

This is an ancient form of divination for which most naturists or witches were charged with during the period of the burnings. On a windy day go deep into a forestry where you will not be disturbed. Lie down among the trees selecting a patch where the trees are particularly leafy. Relax and close your eyes and feel mother earth underneath you.

When you are completely relaxed you can concentrate on the wind rustling through the leafy trees. Scientists have tried to capture the voices that they themselves have heard however even with modern day technology, they have been unable to do so.

The voices that you hear are messages far beyond your conscious mind and are very relevant for you. Listen carefully and you will be surprised at what you may hear. Never fear the whispering wind.

Healing Animals

An ancient remedy to heal an animal with an open wound is to gather four red thistle blooms before daybreak. You then put one bloom each on the four points of the compass, North, South, East and West and place a stone in the centre. You take the wounded animal and place it on the stone and leave for several minutes. The reason for this is that the power of the spell is in the thistle which is a wonderful vitalising plant. The four flowers which are placed at each point North, South, East and West, directs the power of the thistle directly into the animal. When the animal recovers place a sachet of rue around its neck to ward off illness.

Fertility Charms

If you wish to increase your fertility carry a small sachet of hazelnuts. Other herbs used to increase fertility include, poppy, cucumber, apple, acorns, myrtle and hazel. For men they should carry a sachet of mandrake root to increase their fertility. Men can also carry acorns to increase their fertility rate.

Marriage Charms

On a Friday during a waxing moon select 10 dried yarrow flower heads. You bind all of the stems together and tie a small green ribbon bow around them. Hang it over the maritial bed to avoid fighting or confrontation.

End of Love

If you wish to end a relationship or your lover leaves you carry one of these herbs to ease the pain; Balm of Gilead or Valerian. Alternatively, if you are feeling hurt just inhale freshly grounded rue leaves. To completely forget a lover just carry a sachet of this mixture; Honeysuckle, Chichory and Purslane.

Love Potions

On a Friday night as the moon is waxing gather some orris root and mix with olive oil in an earthware container. Place the bowl on your table and say: *'Love, Love, Love, Love, Love, Love, Love (seven times)'*. Pour the oil into a dark bottle and close tightly. On the following Friday night open the bottle anytime from then after. The oil can be worn by the person at any time needed.

Flying Ointments

C AUTION: Only to be used by the very experienced.

Herbs: Aconite, Foxglove and Water Parsnip.

Mix the three herbs above. First you must shread them, then grind them into a powder form and seep them in pig's lard or some fat similar. Rub the ointment onto your body whilst kneeling down beside a fire. It is said that your physical body remains beside the fire for warmth and your astral body leaves to wander outer plains.

Other herbs which can be used for flying or out of body experiences include Basil, Cinquefoil, Parlsey, Sunflower Seeds and Sweet Flag.

This procedure should be done by a highly experienced herbalist or witch as the results can be fatal.

Superstitions

Some of the enclosed superstitions are old wive's tales, witches knowledge and general superstitions handed down through the ages. They are many and varied and are listed in alphabetical order.

AFTERBIRTH: The afterbirth (placenta) is known to have magical properties. One of the oldest superstitions associated with afterbirth is when you burn it you count the number of pops that it makes and that is considered how long the child shall live.

AMBER: This semi-precious stone has been used for generations to ward off evil and witchcraft. It has been worn as an amulet and is particularly useful for new born babies.

ANGELICA: This plant is cooked and used for protection against rabies, plague and other serious illnesses.

ASHES: The cold ashes of a fire are still used today by many cultures. They are mainly used as a fertility charm and rubbed externally on the body.

BATCHELOR'S BUTTONS: This is a small button type flower (somewhat like a buttercup). It was once used by young single men to fortell their future love.

BAT: The appearance of a bat in a church during a wedding is considered a very bad omen. If a bat hits a house or windowpane it means impending death of someone who lives there.

BEARDS: Having a beard is considered unchristian. Men with beards are not to be trusted and if you have a red beard you are very dishonest.

BEDWETTING: To stop a child bedwetting (or an adult) you burn a mouse and serve it to the person within a pie.

BIRTHMARK: If a child is born with a birthmark superstition says that the mother was exposed to a dreadful fright or evil.

CANDLE: If you have difficulty lighting a candle it signifies rain is imminent. The only time you can leave candles burn alone in an empty room is on Christmas Eve which brings prosperity.

CATS: A cat is perceived to have the most supernatural powers and this is why it is identified with witchcraft. A sneezing cat promises rain. A cat that sits with its back to a fire knows that there is a storm on the way.

CHARM: A charm can be made up of many things that have magical powers. A prayer, a saying or a sachet can ward off evil. Good luck charms are still common in everyday use such as 'bless you' when a person coughs or sneezes.

CLOVER: This is considered to be the best form of good luck, a four leaved clover. It is said to bring tremendous luck and ward off evil.

DAISY: This tiny little plant is known for the ritual of pulling out the leaves 'He loves me, he loves me not'. If you place a daisy under your pillow at night your true love will come to you in your dreams.

DOGS: A dalmation is considered a very lucky dog. If a dog scratches himself and is tired it is a sign that there is going to be a change in the weather. A dog that howls at night and comes back to howl on a second night signifies death within the house.

DRUNK: There are many ancient cures for a drunkard one being to mix the persons blood with owl eggs and the powder of dead mans bones.

DUNG: Poultices are still made today in many cultures from the dung of an Ox which has tremendous healing powers. Stepping in dog dirt is highly lucky.

EAGLE: These tremendous birds are linked with strength and power. Seeing a few eagles flying together is a sign of peace.

EARTHQUAKE: All animals know when an earthquake is coming as their behaviour changes as they seek cover or try to warn humans about the upcoming event. Earthquakes have many and varied superstitions around them and are generally associated with great fear.

ECLIPSE: For generations people have lived in great fear of an Eclipse. It is thought that during an eclipse evil spirits roam and try to take over your body.

EYEBROW: The shape of your eyebrows determines what kind of person you are. If a man's eyebrows join you are not to be trusted, if a woman's eyebrows join it is a sure sign of a happy marriage.

FLEAS: It is an old supersticion that when it is going to rain that fleas bite you more. The only way to rid yourself of fleas is by jumping through a large fire at midnight on the night of the Summer Solstice.

FLYING OINTMENT: So many people used to think that flying ointment was made up of babies fat and the blood of rats.

FOX: The fox throughout generations has been known as a sly animal and associated with evil. If a fox comes near your home it signifies a disaster.

FUNERAL: A coffin should always leave the dead person's house by the front door as if it does not it means they may have trouble getting to the afterlife. At the funeral itself all mourners must ensure not to walk in front of the coffin or block it's departure in any way into the new world.

GARLIC: A well known enemy of Vampires and witchcraft. However, in herbalism garlic is a great against fighting worms, illness and earache.

GHOSTS: Whether human or animal are greatly feared when they return to earth. Peoples fears include their return for revenge or as a warning.

GORSE: This is considered an unlucky bush and contains hostility. If you bring gorse bushes into your home you are inviting death.

GRAVES: During burial a body must be laid facing east-west. If you drop something into an open grave accidentally other than a flower or earth you invite death onto yourself.

HATS: If you put your hat on the wrong way around you will have bad luck for the day.

HEADACHE: The most bizzard cure for a headache is to get moss from a deadman's skull and inhale it.

HENBANE: Due to it very poisonous make-up henbane is one of the most used during witchcraft.

HORSE: The horse is one of the more magical animals. One even etched into a mountainside in England. Horses are supposed to be able to see ghosts.

INITIALS: Anybody who's initials of their name spell out a work is considered very lucky.

IRON: If you want evil or a witch to stop entering your home place something iron under or at your doorstep.

IVORY: Ivory is thought to ward off cancer.

IVY: This is a very special plant. It is a protector against evil and it can cure rashes.

JACKDAW: They are considered to be very bad omens. It is very unlucky to see a jackdaw on it's own.

JADE: This gemstone is considered very lucky in the far east. It was used to cure spleen problems

JAUNDICE: Remedies for the cure of jaundice include spreading ten lice on bread and butter and eating it.

JUNIPER: This is a very sacred and holy magical bush. It is used for protection and for treating epilepsy.

KISS: A kiss is a wonderful sign of effection and loyalty. Kiss amulets signify good fortune.

KNEE: If you have an itchy knee it means that you are very jealous of someone.

KNIFE: On a table knives should not be allowed to cross each other as this is very unfornutate for the person who allows it to happen.

KNOT: Knots are known as magical in the nautical world. If you want to get a look at your future husband tie 7 knots in your garter and place under your pillow.

LAME: If you come across a lame person or animal it is extremely unlucky.

LAUGHS: Ancient superstition thought that if a baby laughed you must immediately make the sign of the cross on their mouth to ward off evil spirits entering their souls.

LEAP YEARS: If you have a good idea the best time to try for it is during a leap year.

LETTER: If two letters cross in the post this is extremy unlucky.

MAKE-UP: It is very unlucky on opening night for an actor or actress to spill their face powder.

MARIGOLD: For generations this flower has been used as an aphrodisiac. If you want to cure a headache just smell a marigold.

MAYDAY: Was and still is considered the most magical day other than the solstices. On the first day of May sprinkle fresh flowers on your doorstep to bring health, wealth and happiness into the house for the coming year.

MIRRORS: We all know the saying if you break a mirror you will get 'seven years bad luck'. Other superstitions say that if you look into a mirror at midnight that has a candle lighting on both sides, you will see the face of the devil.

NAMES: Every name has its own qualities including magical. Never name a baby after another child in the house who has died.

NIGHTENGALE: An ancient English lore believes that if you hear a nightengale sings before the Cuckoo that love is imminent.

NIGHTSHADE: This is yet another favourite for the use in spells by witches'. It is yet another ingredient that can be introduced into flying ointment.

NUTMEG: This is considered to be a very lucky spice and if you sprinkle it onto your Bingo or Lottery card...you never know.

OAK: This is the most powerful of trees and is magical. Never take shelter under an oak during a thunderstorm.

OLIVE: This tree is renowned for serenity. Therefore, it wards off all evil and witchcraft.

ONYX: This gemstone is associates with witchcraft. It was widely used for death spells, it can bring on nightmares and insomnia.

ORANGES: This fruit is great for fertility and lovers should exchange an orange as a gift when they get engaged.

PANSY: The pansy must not be picked during good weather as this will draw up a storm.

PARSLEY: Have you ever heard that 'only the wicked grow parsley' or 'a witch must have parsley growing by her gate'? Parsley is associated with evil however if you are suffering from nausea and carry it, the nausea will subside.

PEARLS: The pearl is the birthstone of June to a baby ensures a long and healthy life.

PEONY: This flower is known for healing and if you wear a necklace made from the roots it can relieve epilepsy.

QUAIL: Eggs from the quail are renouned for prosperity and wealth.

RAINBOW: In many cultures if a rainbow arches over a house this means a death will follow very soon.

RAVEN: This bird for generations has been associated with witchcraft and is an omen of bad luck.

ROSE: The flower of love. If you send your lover a red rose it signifies lust, desire and passion. If you send your lover a white rose it signifies commitment and true love.

RUBY: Is the birthstone for the month of July. It is considered a very lucky stone and will keep you safe from all evil. It is said that a ruby on your finger will change colour depending on your health.

SALT: Since salt was discovered it is considered magical. It is still used today in Christian baptisms or if you think a fire may be used for the purpose of witchcraft just sprinkle salt onto it.

SAPPHIRE: Is the birthstone for September. In Buddhism the Sapphire has very special powers and is greatly revered.

SEAGULL: Within the nautical world the Seagull is considered very unlucky. It is also widely believed that if you see a seagull over land that a storm will shortly follow.

SKULLS: The human skull has been used in many rituals and is considered to possess great magical powers. Scorcerers focus on the human skull as the seat of the soul.

THATCH: A very old ritual is if you believe that a witch has put a curse on you steal some of the thatch from her roof and this will break the hex.

THIRTEEN: Amost everyone is aware that this number is supposed to be unlucky. Hotels will not have a floor thirteen and even today some streets will be notibly missing a house number thirteen.

TOAD: Like the cat this is another animal associated with witchcraft. The poor toad was almost part of every spell and due to the association with a witch were frequently spat on or killed.

TRUNKS: Old travelling trunks should never ever be locked if the owner is away. Today this is still used frequently in seafaring families.

UMBILICAL CORD: It is said that if you burn the unbilical cord the baby that it belongs to will die by fire. If you throw it into the sea the baby will drown. Never give an unbilical cord to a witch as they may be able to take over the babies soul.

UNICORN: This is the most magical of all horses. Only a pure virgin can capture a Unicorn.

VIOLET: These beautiful flowers should never be brought inside your house as they will bring you extreme bad luck.

VIRGINITY: As above, only virgins can catch a unicorn. You can find out if a girl is a virgin if she forgets to put the salt cellar on the table or if you put a small piece of coaldust into her food she will want to go to the bathroom regularly.

WARTS: The array of treatments for warts goes from the bizzare to the extremely bizzare. If you mix holy water and the blood of a pig this will cure warts. You can also spit on them each morning when you awake or whenever there is a full moon.

WEDDING CAKE: Your wedding cake should be very rich in flavour which will bring you wealth in your future marriage. If a bride retains a slice of her wedding cake her husband shall always remain faithful.

A Herbal Wheel or Garden

A herbal garden is a must if you wish to have fresh produce at your fingertips. You can either grow your herbs in a herbal wheel, in containers or directly into the earth. Decide what herbs you are most interested in growing and start off limiting the amount of herbs grown. Your garden (or wheel) may be laid out in accordance of the requirements of the particular plants e.g, Mint is best kept in a container as it will take over your garden. Just use your imagination and you can form a mini work-of-wonder with rocks, water and herbs. Choose a pattern, select the herbs according to their conditions (sun, shade etc.) and decide on where you are going to position them.

The land should be fertile and nobody should intefere with your herbs. You then plant your herbs during the waxing moon or plant when the moon is in Cancer, Pisces, Taures and Capricorn. To protect your herb garden plant four red plants such as roses or geraniums as this keeps away evil spirits. When your garden ready and you have an abundance of fresh herbs remember to always ask permission of the plant before to take any foliage away from it.

\#

A HEALING GARDEN: You will need to plant garlic, onion, carnations, rosemary, sage, peppermint, rue and wood sorrell.

A LOVE GARDEN: You will need to plant the old variety of roses, yarrow, lavender, basil, violets, vervian, lemon balm and loveage.

A DIVINATION GARDEN: You will need to plant yarrow, borage, mugworth, wormword, cinquefoil, anise and lavender.

A herbal wheel can be easily constructed out of about thirty small bricks. You start on the outer circle and build upwards until you reach the apex. Then you fill in with good clean soil and plant according to the herb's requirements. This takes up about three feet and is about three feet in height. A cost-effective and attractive alternative if you do not have a large garden.

Contacts
BOOKS OF INTEREST

KARMA by ROCHELLE MOORE -

This book can be ordered on Amazon.com or directly through Kashmir International, Rockbrook House, Blackrock, Co Dublin, Ireland. (Fax: 00353 1 2883243)
or by contacting Rochelle at Rochelle.Moore@hotmail.com. Karma is a book that introduces you to a new and more positive way of life. It looks at various aspects of religion, psychological negativity and offeres an array of how to move forward and change your world for the better.

AROMA SCIENCE by DR MARIA LIS-BALCHIN -

This book contains a list of oils and scientific analysis. It includes sections on metodology and the sense of smell. It can be ordered online.

NATURE'S HERB COMPANY -

Suppies dried herbs and a full catalogue of herbs. They can be reached at 281 Ellis Street, San Francisco, CA 94102.

About the Author

Rochelle Moore is a published writer, a poet, loves nature, aromatherapy and natural remedies. To date Rochelle has published many insightful poems, short stories, a book about Karma and she is now concentrating on writing about natural thearapies. All the recipes in this book are easy to follow and can be used at home.

Rochelle lives in Ireland and loves all aspects of nature, animal rescue, Karma and horses. She is a spirual person who believes in the good nature of most people. This book is written for those who would like to experiment at home with aromatherapy and ancient herbal recipes. If this book had have been written a couple of hundred years ago, Rochelle would have been burned at the stake for using nature's own sources to heal and improve many aspect of your lives.

While the author has made every possible effort to ensure that the contents of this book are accurate, it is not to be regarded as a substitute for professional medical advice. Neither the author nor the publishers can accept any legal responsibility for any problems with the readers health which results in the use of self-help described within this book. Oils and herbs are very potent and this easy-to-use book provides an alternative form of life. If your symptoms persist please contact your doctor or a medical professional immediately.

The oils and herbs used in this book are easily obtained. They can be purchased in stores, grown in the wild, grown in a herbal wheel in your garden or ordered online. This book brings you step-by-step through the many processes of drying herbs and oils and for treating many physical and psychological ailments.